Th

PALEO BREAKTHROUGH™

A Revolutionary Protocol to Rapidly Decrease Inflammation and Balance Your Immune System

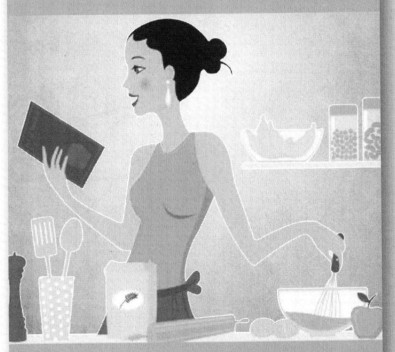

by Anne Angelone, Licensed Acupuncturist

THE AUTOIMMUNE PALEO BREAKTHROUGH

A Revolutionary Protocol to Rapidly Decrease Inflammation and Balance Your Immune System

by

Anne Angelone

Copyright © by Anne Angelone 2013

All Rights Reserved

ISBN-13: 9781493688814 ISBN-10 1493688812

Image Credit: with permission from 123RF.com

To request permission for reproduction or to inquire about consulting for autoimmunity, please contact:

Anne Angelone, Licensed Acupuncturist

website: www.paleobreakthrough.com

Table of Contents

PREFACE

Welcome to *The Autoimmune Paleo Breakthrough*. In this book, I provide a much-needed method for effectively treating autoimmune disease. For those readers familiar with the Paleo autoimmune protocol, this method combines an advanced version of this dietary template with sound principles of Functional Medicine to give patients (and health care practitioners) a fundamental guide for successfully treating autoimmune disease.

The Autoimmune Paleo Breakthrough establishes the Paleo autoimmune protocol as the cornerstone of an effective DIY (do-it-yourself) dietary plan that patients can use to treat autoimmune disease. The Paleo autoimmune protocol I present here consists of an advanced elimination diet that has been shown to accelerate immune balance faster than diets commonly suggested by many practitioners (such as the grain- and nightshade-filled elimination diets).

In addition to using this advanced Paleo autoimmune protocol, I also discuss the critical importance of applying Functional Medicine principles to treat autoimmune reactions and inflammation. By Functional Medical principles, I am referring to the following types of treatments:

- removing triggers
- treating the root causes while prioritizing healing intestinal permeability
- balancing the immune system
- supporting detoxification and methylation
- clearing infections

It's my belief that practitioners of all types of medicine, including Traditional, Integrative, Western, and Functional Medicine, can use this method to treat patients with autoimmune disease. In terms of a patient's overall health, this is the most efficient way to dramatically reduce the immune/inflammatory response that causes a wide range of symptoms in those suffering from autoimmune disease.

There are no easy answers when it comes to treating autoimmune disease. And there's certainly no one-size-fits-all solution. That's why, in my opinion, the future of effective treatment for each patient must be based on applying a personalized version of the protocol described in this book, along with natural medicine, to maintain a balanced, healthy immune system.

One of my primary recommendations in this book is to ensure that patients and practitioners clearly understand the foods to avoid when treating autoimmune disease. These activating foods include grains, dairy, soy, eggs, nightshades, nuts, seeds, and certain oils and spices. You'll find these items described in detail throughout the book and listed in the "Foods to Include and Eliminate" section of this book.

I also believe that patients and practitioners need to take a close look at all of the seemingly "safe natural medicines" that are available today and closely scrutinize labels for immune stimulating herbs that can actually cause more harm than good for patients suffering from autoimmune disease.

So, once again, welcome to *The Autoimmune Paleo Breakthrough*. After years of treating patients with a wide variety of autoimmune conditions, I have written this book with the sincere hope that it serves as a useful guide for anyone seeking effective solutions for treating autoimmune disease.

INTRODUCTION

If you're reading this book, it's probably because you've suffered from an autoimmune condition for months or even years, and you know from personal experience that certain foods contribute to your condition.

Like most of us with the same condition, you've already tried the conventional medical approach for treating your autoimmune disease, but you're still struggling with the pain, fatigue, digestive problems, inflammation, and even depression caused by most autoimmune conditions. And, quite frankly, you're more than ready for change.

As you've looked harder for solutions, you've probably already noticed that patients who've been following the Paleo autoimmune protocol know more than the average health care provider about why this protocol, or dietary template, has been so successful.

We know, for example, that certain foods, toxins, and herbs irritate the immune system. And scientific literature has demonstrated that a range of medical problems, including nutrient deficiencies, intestinal permeability (commonly known as leaky gut), methylation defects, and genetic variations, are specific to autoimmune disease.

In addition, we know that many factors, such as chronic stress, intestinal permeability (leaky gut), infections, poor sleep, and malnutrition, can cause immunological imbalance. To put it in more technical terms, each of these factors can contribute to a failure of regulatory T-cells (i.e., the cells that balance your immune system) and cytokine dysregulation (i.e., the cells that make you feel inflamed), which ultimately results in autoimmune disease.

The good news is that the research linking autoimmunity to these health problems is starting to reach the mainstream.

The bad news, however, is that this information has not yet thoroughly or consistently reached all of the health practitioners treating patients suffering from autoimmune disease. Many primary care physicians, rheumatologists, and alternative care providers still don't have the latest information about autoimmunity.

Fortunately, *The Autoimmune Paleo Breakthrough* provides you with a variety of options for taking charge of your autoimmune well-being.

The Autoimmune Paleo Breakthrough consists of a simple yet profound do-it-yourself (DIY) plan for treating the majority of autoimmune conditions. By following the guidance provided in this book, you have everything you need to take an active role in treating your autoimmune disease—and even getting to a point where the disease goes into remission. Of course we have to face the fact that there is no cure for autoimmune disease i.e. once your genes are turned on, they never turn off. The good news is that your inflammatory gene expression can be "dimmed down" to the point where your symptoms disappear, which is the goal of *The Autoimmune Paleo Breakthrough.* This is a radical shift from the typical solutions we've heard to date, which usually run along the lines of "just learn to live with it" or "let's bombard it with steroids."

Those responses to autoimmune disease, which don't do anything to address the underlying problem of the disease, represent the old model. It's time now to actively embrace the new model—and that's exactly what you can do with this book.

How does it work? In *The Autoimmune Paleo Breakthrough*, you'll learn how you can adjust your diet to calm inflammation naturally, while also learning how to investigate and correct the root causes of your autoimmune reactions. In terms of your daily routine, you'll be empowered to affect change three or more times a day by feeding your body the right kinds of food for optimal immune cell function.

The dietary template provided in this book is designed to rapidly reduce inflammation and heal intestinal permeability (leaky gut). To calm down your immune/inflammatory response and allow your gut to heal, you'll need to remove the major offending foods (including eggs, grains, alcohol, nightshades, nuts, seeds, legumes, and dairy) for at least 30 days.

Some patients do really well on this protocol in less than 30 days; others choose to stay committed to it for several months to one year or even longer. No matter how long you're on the plan, the goal is ultimately twofold. First, the protocol aims to increase anti-inflammatory and probiotic foods, which in turn heal the integrity of the gut lining. Secondly, the protocol eliminates the foods that create a low-grade immune/inflammatory response, irritate the gut lining, or nurture harmful bacteria. By following this dietary plan, you can eventually eliminate the underlying causes of inflammation and autoimmunity and balance your overactive immune system.

The book includes a "Foods to Include and Eliminate" section as well as delicious and easy-to-make Paleo recipes to help you keep your dietary plan on track. You'll also find a resource section for websites and other books containing more information (and more Paleo recipes).

In addition to learning about foods to include in your diet (and irritating foods to avoid), you will be introduced to some other important considerations when it comes to treating autoimmune disease. These considerations include:

- resolving gastrointestinal infections
- balancing the immune system
- supporting detoxification
- reducing stress
- increasing glutathione
- increasing regulatory T-cells

You may find all of this to be very daunting, especially if you don't have a health care background. But gaining an understanding of the material in this book is critical to unlocking the clues for treating your autoimmune condition. Keep in mind that treating your condition shouldn't be a solo project; it's very important to work with a health care practitioner who has experience with autoimmune disease and in interpreting the tests you'll need to take to uncover the drivers of your autoimmune disease.

There's no doubt that following the protocol outlined in *The Autoimmune Paleo Breakthrough* takes a serious level of commitment. No cheating allowed! But by following the protocol for 30 days, your immune system will be shored up with the right nutrition, which in turn will help your inflamed gut begin to heal and your immune system to come back into balance.

Remember, the goal here is to treat your autoimmune disease (in particular by fixing your leaky gut). And your best chance for doing this is to eliminate all triggers to autoimmune reactions. This, in turn, will decrease your flare-ups and the severity of autoimmune attacks. Patients who follow this protocol admit that it can be tough. They also come to recognize and appreciate the overall health benefits that come with sticking to the plan and making it work.

RAISING THE BAR FOR IMMUNE SYSTEM BALANCE: A NEW CLINICAL MODEL FOR AUTOIMMUNE DISEASE

TREATING AUTOIMMUNE DISEASE WITH AUTOIMMUNE PALEO NUTRITION AND FUNCTIONAL MEDICINE

We're currently witnessing an evolutionary shift in chronic disease management, particularly for autoimmune disease. Patients have been demanding a new model that moves away from the "disease-care" management of symptoms and instead provides investigative medicine that treats the root causes of disease.

The American Autoimmune Related Disease Association (AARDA) calculates that 1 in 12 women and 1 in 25 men in the United States have an autoimmune disease. Moreover, more than 50 million Americans have at least one autoimmune disease, according to AARDA. Even more astounding is the fact that more Americans suffer from autoimmune disease than they do from cancer and heart disease combined.

These statistics don't even reflect the fact that many patients suffer from "silent autoimmunity" (i.e., they have symptoms of an autoimmune disease but no tissue destruction) for ten years before they're actually diagnosed with an autoimmune condition, which generally comes only after tissues are destroyed. This astounding trend needs to change. Indeed, it can change because we now know more than ever about the underlying triggers causing autoimmune disease. Read on to learn about the underlying mechanisms that trigger autoimmune disease and how you can combat them with the Paleo autoimmune protocol and Functional Medicine.

"Paleo" is the term used by those who follow the diet of our pre-agricultural ancestors. The Paleo diet is free of all the grains, processed foods, and sugars that are consumed by the majority of people today. The standard Paleo dietary template has received merit because it consists of the right food choices for reversing many common chronic diseases in the modern world. When you follow the Paleo lifestyle, you receive the benefits of eating the right foods; you also are encouraged to get adequate sleep, sunlight, exercise, and relaxation for optimal health, disease prevention, and even remission.

There is abundant research available today suggesting the benefit of adopting a nutrient-dense ancestral diet as a template for preventing and even reversing all types of chronic disease. Paleo scientists, Functional Medicine practitioners, anthropologists, MD internists, psychiatrists, biochemistry professors, patients, gym owners, bloggers recounting their own Paleo experiences, and others have been taking the same basic message about Paleo into the mainstream. That message is to eat only what your ancestral genes can recognize, and thrive on nutrient-dense protein, good fats, and plants, while simultaneously avoiding the environmental inputs of disease expression (including sugar, grain, and hydrogenated veggie oils).

While there's an ever-increasing amount of information available about the underlying causes of autoimmune disease, research tends to precede the actual practice of mainstream medicine by about ten years. So, in all likelihood your rheumatologist or other medical practitioner doesn't know much if anything about the association of intestinal permeability with autoimmune disease unless they read the latest PubMed papers or attend Functional Medicine conferences or The Ancestral Health Symposium. Nor will they be familiar with the latest information for treating autoimmune disease with dietary intervention.

The Autoimmune Paleo Breakthrough provides you with critical information about the underlying causes of autoimmune disease and guidance in following a complete anti-inflammatory dietary template. This dietary plan focuses on increasing nutrient density from plants and animals while avoiding harmful triggers, such as eggs, grains, alcohol, nightshades, seeds, nuts, seed- and nightshade-based spices, seed-based oils, immune stimulating herbs, legumes, and dairy. All of these foods have been shown to be the worst triggers of leaky gut.

Many who've followed a standard Paleo diet to combat autoimmune disease have found they have to tailor their diet a bit further beyond the standard Paleo template to more effectively treat their condition. That's why the advanced autoimmune protocol presented in this book does go further than the basic Paleo protocol to halt autoimmune reactions.

FUNCTIONAL MEDICINE

Functional Medicine is a medical approach that focuses on treating the underlying mechanisms of disease. This approach is fast becoming the new lens through which patients and practitioners can collaborate to treat and modulate immune responses. Practitioners of Functional Medicine treat autoimmune disease and balance the immune system by using a variety of techniques, including the autoimmune Paleo dietary protocol, the 4R program (described below), and safe natural medicine protocols.

In my practice as a licensed acupuncturist and Functional Medicine practitioner, I tell my patients that Functional Medicine is Chinese Medicine plus lab testing. Functional Medicine follows the philosophy of restoring organ function that is a cornerstone of Chinese Medicine while also incorporating the latest scientific research about how our genetics, environment, and lifestyle all interact and affect our health.

Patients with autoimmune diseases tend to suffer from a range of root-cause conditions, including blood sugar imbalance, hidden infection, methylation defects, dysbiosis, and specific vitamin and enzyme deficiencies. Because of these underlying problems, patients must often go beyond the Paleo autoimmune food protocol and may need to consider additional methods for treating the underlying contributors to their autoimmune disease. A qualified practitioner of Functional Medicine can help guide you through the appropriate testing for getting to the bottom of your autoimmune condition.

THE 4 R PROGRAM AND THE PALEO AUTOIMMUNE PROTOCOL

In my own practice, I routinely order lab work to test for a wide range of potential triggers to autoimmune disease. I also apply the Paleo autoimmune protocol along with acupuncture and the 4 R program described below to dramatically alter the course of autoimmune conditions.

Developed by Jeffrey Bland, the 4 R program (Remove, Replace, Re-inoculate, and Repair) recognizes that most inflammation comes from the gut. The goals of the 4 R program, which has been the mainstay of Functional Medicine for treating all chronic and inflammatory illnesses, are similar to the goals of the Paleo autoimmune protocol, which is why these two methods work so well together.

Let's take a quick look at the 4 R program and how each of the four "R's" compare to stages in the Paleo autoimmune protocol.

"Remove" means removing toxins in foods, irritants to the gut lining, food allergies, food sensitivities, yeast, bacteria, and parasites. In the Paleo autoimmune protocol, this is the equivalent to the elimination phase of the diet. This would be a good time in your treatment to consider working with a Functional Medicine practitioner to take a stool and blood test.

"Replace" means replacing stomach acid and digestive enzymes. Doing this with food is easy. It is also recommended to add a shot of apple cider vinegar to water at the start of high-protein meals and to include bitter greens (such as arugula and endive) to stimulate your parietal cells to release stomach acid. If this is not enough, hydrochloric acid tablets and digestive enzymes may be helpful.

"Re-inoculate" means restoring beneficial gut flora. Many Functional Medicine practitioners suggest beneficial probiotic supplements to replenish normal gut flora. This is the equivalent of adding fermented foods as suggested in the Paleo autoimmune protocol.

"Repair" means supplying nutrients to heal the mucosal lining of the gut and support the gut's immune function. This echoes the recommendation by followers of the Paleo autoimmune protocol to utilize bone broths and organ meats. This soothes and heals the gut lining while also supplying adequate nutrition for efficient immune function. This specific recommendation may be adequate for many patients; others, however, may need to add glutamine, zinc l-carnosine, glycine, and DGL to receive the full benefit.

Functional Medicine practitioners who've been applying the treatment principles of the 4 R program have witnessed their patients getting better quickly. Testing for food sensitivities, leaky gut, cross-reactive proteins, blood sugar imbalance, anemia, vitamin D deficiencies, adrenal fatigue, methylation defects, auto-antibodies, and gastro-intestinal and other infections has become one of the most efficient ways to investigate the underlying causes of autoimmune disease.

NUTRITIONAL EPIGENOMICS

Nutritional epigenomics aka Nutrigenomics, is the exciting field of study that looks at how food and nutrients can regulate inflammatory gene expression and thus suppress the inflammatory response. Researchers have found that certain nutrients can flip the switch on certain genes, turning them either on or off. The more technical term for silencing inflammatory gene suppression via certain nutrients is DNA methylation. Research shows that proper methylation can be aided by taking adequate amounts of folate, vitamin B6, and vitamin B12.

Functional Medicine practitioners use nutritional epigenomics to treat chronic disease. In fact, many of the concepts of nutritional epigenomics are similar to what you find in the Paleo autoimmune protocol. According to the practitioners of nutritional epigenomics, we need to eat in ways that allow the best possible genetic expression. Our genes are much more suited to nutrient-dense, unprocessed whole foods versus having to contend with the triggers found in modern processed foods that continually fire the immune/inflammatory response.

For anyone suffering from autoimmune disease, the primary goal of treatment is to suppress the inflammatory response. If we know how to turn off the inflammatory response at the level of our genes (i.e., by feeding exactly the right nutrition to the epigenome, which is the area just above the genes and where an exchange of nutrients can occur), we can affect the best possible genetic expression and therefore have a healthier, less inflamed life.

Nutritional epigenomics also considers genetic variations like mutations and slight receptor site defects on our genes, which are called Single Nucleotide Polymorphisms (SNPs), that may require higher doses of certain nutrients or vitamins (such as vitamin D). As it turns out, SNPs are common in patients with autoimmune disease and there are tests to find out what your particular SNP's are and specific supplementation that may be helpful. One helpful lab is 23andMe.

As researchers continue to uncover specific nutritional deficiencies along with likely SNPs, we will even more fully understand the importance of nutrient density in immune function and the appropriate therapeutic dosing requirements beyond dietary intervention.

Since the Paleo autoimmune template encourages nutrient-dense organic greens, organ meats, and pastured meats, it's a great starting point for adding more of these methylation factors into your diet. Some patients may also need to consider supplementing the basic Paleo diet with other important methylation factors. By finding the right combination of anti-inflammatory foods and supplements that help combat inflammation, you may be able to safely and effectively quiet down and perhaps even put your disease into remission. It's been known to work!

FIVE QUICK TIPS FOR HALTING AUTOIMMUNE REACTIONS

Patients seeking to halt autoimmune reactions must be able to do the following five things very well:

1. Identify and remove your dietary, environmental, and emotional stress triggers.
2. Actively work on healing your leaky gut.
3. Silence your inflammatory gene expression.
4. Build up your regulatory T-cells.
5. Replenish your glutathione and micronutrient deficiencies.

Finding the right health care practitioner is a critical part of ensuring that you can stay on track with these five important steps.

AUTOIMMUNE TRIGGERS

The significant increase of autoimmune disease is no doubt due to the dramatic increase of modern environmental triggers (i.e., immune activating foods and chemicals) that lead to barrier system permeability (most notably leaky gut) and set the stage for a range of autoimmune conditions. When it comes to autoimmune disease, it is clear that dietary toxins are the biggest environmental triggers for intestinal permeability.

For anyone with an autoimmune disease, the first steps are to eliminate all known inflammatory foods, resolve dysbiosis and SIBO (you can find out more about these conditions later in the book), clear infections, and heal the mucosal lining of the small intestine (i.e., healing your leaky gut). All of this will go a long way to reducing inflammation and balancing the immune system.

In addition to diet, and depending on how you react to initial treatment, you may also want to monitor other significant promoters of autoimmune disease, including environmental toxins, stress, lack of sleep, disruption of circadian rhythms, poor digestion, infections, hormonal imbalances, blood sugar dysregulation, and micronutrient deficiencies.

LEAKY GUT?
WHAT DOES THAT MEAN?

Intestinal permeability (or leaky gut) refers to the opening of the mucosal lining in the small intestine that allows food, yeast, and bacteria in the intestines to interact with the immune system. Current discoveries in the field of immunity confirm that certain foods and bacteria irritate the mucosal lining of the gut and contribute both to intestinal permeability (leaky gut) and the autoimmune response, which most patients generally experience as a flare-up, attack, or an exacerbation of symptoms.

As you start to look into the causes of your autoimmune condition, you'll be tasked with looking through a new lens to consider how poorly digested foods continue to irritate the lining of your gut, feed yeast and bacterial overgrowths, and trigger autoantibody responses. Since 80% of the immune system is located in the gut, you should know, if you don't already, that digestive health is of paramount importance when it comes to treating and healing autoimmune disease.

While your doctor may not have heard of it, leaky gut has been associated with autoimmune disease, and identified in scientific literature, for many years. What's exciting now is that we are starting to get a better understanding about how leaky gut is the way through which our genes and foods/toxins can interact to set off autoimmune reactions.

While leaky gut has been on the radar of "integrative medicine" practitioners since the early 1990s, it's just now starting, finally, to become a household term because of the recent scientific validation of intestinal permeability as an underlying prerequisite for the autoantibody reaction to occur in Celiac disease. To put it another way, it's only through leaky gut that environmental triggers (e.g. in this case gluten) can interact with our genes. This new information broadens the consideration of leaky gut as a prerequisite for all autoimmune disease reactions to occur. According to Dr. Alessio Fasano of the Maryland Center for Celiac Research, leaky gut may play a significant role in triggering most autoimmune conditions.

Intestinal permeability has been found in cases of every autoimmune disease that have been investigated so far (which is about 30%).

Leaky gut has been found in the following autoimmune diseases: Ankylosing Spondylitis, Apthous stomatitis, autism, autoimmune gastritis, autoimmune hepatitis, Behcet's Syndrome, Celiac disease, Depression, Dermatitis Herpetiformis, Type 1 Diabetes, Eczema, gut migraine in children, and Hashimoto's Thyroiditis. Leaky gut is also frequently found in cases of asthma, psoriasis, and nearly all of the idiopathic juvenile arthritides.

Taking into account the growing amount of research that shows the connection between leaky gut and autoimmune disease, healing a leaky gut may prove to be the single biggest key for halting the progression of autoimmunity.

HOW DO I KNOW IF I HAVE LEAKY GUT SYNDROME?

These days you can do a blood test through a company called Cyrex Labs to find out if you have leaky gut. There are also some obvious signs of leaky gut, including gas, bloating, poor digestion, multiple food and chemical sensitivities, gut pain, and inflammation. Some not-so-obvious signs of leaky gut include decreased mental clarity (often referred to as brain fog), headaches, depression, allergies, eczema, body aches, and fatigue.

Fixing a leaky gut is definitely a priority for anyone suffering from autoimmune disease. Take a look at the following section of the book to see the top triggers of leaky gut so you'll know what to avoid to optimize your gut health and improve your autoimmune condition.

LEAKY GUT TRIGGERS

DIET

Most people blame poor diet as the cause of leaky gut, and rightly so since many popular foods can damage the gut.

Gluten in particular is associated with gut damage.

Other foods contributing to leaky gut include: lectins, which are found in nuts, beans, soy, potatoes, tomatoes, eggplant, peppers, peanut oil, peanut butter, and soy oil as well as other industrial seed oils.

Dairy, saponins, processed foods, excess sugar, alcohol, and fast foods are also common culprits.

MEDICATIONS

The risk of leaky gut can be increased by certain medications, including corticosteroids, antibiotics, antacids, NSAIDS, and some medications for arthritis. Also note that some medications may also contain gluten as filler.

INFECTIONS

An overgrowth of H. pylori (which is a stomach bacteria) can cause leaky gut and ulcers. Overgrowth of other harmful bacteria (SIBO), yeast infections, parasitic infections, and intestinal viruses can also cause leaky gut.

STRESS

Chronic stress raises the adrenal hormone cortisol, which degrades the gut lining and contributes to leaky gut.

HORMONE IMBALANCE

A healthy gut depends on proper hormone levels. Leaky gut can result from deficient or imbalanced estrogen, progesterone, testosterone, or thyroid hormones.

AUTOIMMUNE CONDITIONS

We often think of leaky gut contributing to autoimmune diseases such as Hashimoto's hypothyroidism, rheumatoid arthritis, or psoriasis. While this may be true, other factors can also trigger an autoimmune condition, including toxic exposures or stress. In these cases, managing autoimmunity can be a strategy for improving leaky gut.

INDUSTRIAL FOOD PROCESSING

Leaky gut can be attributed to a variety of methods used by the food processing industry, including the deamidation of wheat to make it water soluble, the high-heat processing (glycation) of sugars, and the addition of excess sugar to processed foods.

VITAMIN D DEFICIENCY

Sufficient vitamin D is vital to good health and helps preserve gut integrity.

POOR GLUTATHIONE STATUS

Glutathione is the body's primary antioxidant and is necessary for defending and repairing the gut lining. Poor diet and lifestyle factors deplete glutathione.

Since these triggers may degrade the mucosal lining of the gut and lead to autoimmune reactions, patients are encouraged to decrease stress, balance their hormones, resolve SIBO and dysbiosis, avoid food sensitivities, and modulate the immune system.

The goal of any treatment plan is always to remove leaky gut triggers, resolve dysbiosis, and restore a healthy intestinal barrier. By doing these things, you are getting yourself on track to reducing any systemic inflammatory reactions that are triggering autoantibody attacks and causing your autoimmune condition.

IMMUNOGENIC OR ALLERGENIC FOOD SENSITIVITIES

If you suffer from an immunogenic reaction to a certain food or foods, it means you are sensitive to the food(s) but not officially allergic. This type of reaction is caused by a low-grade inflammatory response or IgG reaction that activates part of the immune system but does not cause an IgE allergy response or anaphylactic shock.

This type of response in your immune system can be caused by many foods, including gluten, dairy, corn, soy, and nightshade vegetables. With a smoldering and undetected IgG response, along with a leaky gut, your potential for an autoantibody response increases since your immune system is now on high alert to attack the similar protein structures of the offending foods.

ENVIRONMENTAL TOXINS

We are surrounded by toxins in our environment. Some of these toxins have been found to break down immune barriers like the gut. One way to shore up your defense against environmental toxins is to make sure your body has sufficient glutathione, which is the body's primary antioxidant.

We are learning more about how the immune response to chemical exposures can predispose susceptible patients to autoimmune reactions even after the chemical toxin is removed.

From a technical standpoint, this is due to activation of Nuclear Factor Kappa Beta (a potent protein that turns on inflammatory genes). If NFKB is activated, TH17 and IL17 will be activated and inflammation will continue uncontrolled. So, to remedy this immune response to chemical exposures, we can think in terms of an immune equation (> increase TH3, decrease TH17, thereby silencing NFKB for balanced immunity). Basically, this means removing and avoiding the triggers of the TH17 pathway, which also includes chemical exposures.

Besides the foods-to-avoid list and infections, you should also avoid any chemical exposures in your environment; these exposures could include using plastic water bottles that contain bisphenols and sipping out of plastic coffee cup covers.

Also, make sure your food sources are clean and organic, avoid genetically modified foods, hybridized foods, livestock chemicals, toxic cleaning supplies, pharmaceuticals, aflatoxins (mycotoxins) from stored foods, benzenes from cigarette smoke and traffic exhaust, and parabens in makeup, etc.

If you aren't improving on the Paleo food protocol alone, you must consider the possibility that other things, such as the chemical exposures listed here, may be triggering your autoimmune reaction. This is again where it's critical to work with a Functional Medicine practitioner who can order relevant tests from Cyrex Labs.

The following compounds can cause oxidative exposure to the barrier systems in the body, which can in turn lead to a compromised integrity of the lining of the intestines, lungs, and brain.

- Benzene
- Cadmium
- Pesticides
- PCB
- Radiation
- Bisphenol A
- Isocyanates
- Parabens
- Fire Retardants

OTHER SIGNIFICANT TRIGGERS OF INFLAMMATION AND AUTOIMMUNE REACTIONS

SIBO AND DYSBIOSIS

When dealing with an autoimmune condition, it's important to identify and remove overgrowths of yeast, bacteria, and parasites that may also be driving your immune/inflammatory response. By reducing these triggers and fixing the intestinal barrier you will lessen the autoimmune reactions that you may experience outside of the gut (i.e., in the skin, joints, thyroid, and brain).

Dysbiosis refers to an overgrowth of yeast, bacteria, and/or parasites located in the gastrointestinal tract. This generally occurs due to excess sugar and refined carb consumption along with a history of antibiotic use.

Small Intestine Bacterial Overgrowth (SIBO) is now being considered as a significant yet overlooked cause of IBS (Irritable Bowel Syndrome). SIBO can cause nausea, gas, bloating, diarrhea, and/or constipation. Bacterial toxins from SIBO can impair absorption and result in nutrient deficiencies, fat malabsorption, food intolerances, poorly functioning digestive enzymes, leaky gut, and the autoantibody response (i.e., your autoimmune reactions and tissue destruction).

WHAT CAUSES BACTERIAL OVERGROWTH?

The entire gastrointestinal (GI) tract contains bacteria, both good and bad. The small intestine contains bacteria different from that of the large intestine. In the case of SIBO, the small intestine contains too much bacteria that are similar to the ones in the large intestine and should not be living in the small intestine. These bacteria overgrowths then consume sugars and carbohydrates, resulting in a large amounts of gas.

FODMAP malabsorption, inadequate dietary fiber, hypochlorhydria (which is decreased stomach acid), and pancreatic enzyme deficiency set the stage for inadequate digestion in susceptible individuals and contribute to poorly digested carbs, which in turn feed the bacteria in the small intestine. Bacterial endotoxins, called lipopolysaccharides, further contribute to leaky gut and the inflammatory fire that needs to be extinguished in your body.

SIBO DIET

Many people feel better after following a no-starch diet for a month or longer to combat SIBO, though there currently isn't any scientific backing to support this approach. I would recommend starting with autoimmune Paleo diet laid out in this book first. If you still have symptoms that suggest SIBO, then you might consider removing the following starchy veggies for 30 days:

Parsnips, yams, jicama, kohlrabi, okra, sweet potato, taro, plantain, Jerusalem artichoke, parsnips, lotus root, cassava root, manioc, tapioca, yucca.

Others may also need to use antibiotics and/or botanical antimicrobials (dysbiotics) along with extra hydrochloric acid and digestive enzyme supplementation to treat this condition.

Always inform your health care practitioner when you are experiencing these conditions and making these types of dietary changes. If you still have symptoms after trying this approach, you'll need to work with your practitioner to get a definitive test for SIBO or other diagnosis to accurately assess and treat the condition.

RECOVER FASTER: SUPPORT YOUR IMMUNE SYSTEM

GOING BEYOND TH1 AND TH2

When applying the Functional Medicine approach to managing autoimmune disease, we focus on identifying why the immune system is imbalanced and then work to restore that balance. In more scientific terms, we look to balance the two sides of the immune system known as TH1 and TH2.

TH1 is the pro-inflammatory side of the immune system—it responds immediately to an invader into the body. TH2, on the other hand, is the anti-inflammatory side of the immune system. After a delayed response, TH2 produces antibodies to combat an invader. These antibodies tag the invader so that if it shows up again, the immune system can respond more quickly. In a healthy person, these two systems work in balance. In a person suffering from an autoimmune disease, however, one of these systems has become overly dominant.

This imbalance between TH1 and TH2 underlies autoimmune conditions, and we use a safe template like the Paleo autoimmune protocol to help restore balance, tame inflammation, and overcome autoimmune disease.

THE NEW IMMUNE PLAYER: TH17

Recent studies indicate that TH17 is another important player in the immune system. When activated properly, TH17 plays an important role in immune defense. When it over-activates, however, TH17 becomes a factor in autoimmune disease and chronic inflammatory disease.

From a scientific standpoint, TH17 is activated by IL 6, which increases when blood sugar levels drop and when stress responses increase—this includes psychological and emotional stress. When TH17 is activated, it will then amp up IL 17, which activates Nuclear Factor Kappa Beta (NFKB). NFKB is also activated by leaky gut, dysbiosis, SIBO, food sensitivities, stress and viruses. All of this can play a role in triggering autoimmune conditions.

HOW CAN I START DECREASING INFLAMMATION?

Modifying your lifestyle by adopting an advanced Paleo diet is the first step toward decreasing inflammation. Depending on the root cause of your condition, you can also take certain supplements to break the cycle of inflammation and boost your health. Read this section if you want to go deeper into the science of epigenetics for decreasing inflammation.

1. Hack Gene Expression via Methylation

The science of epigenetics basically says that we all come hardwired when it comes to our genomes. While we can't change our genomes, we can change the epigenome (the area just above your genes and where the process of methylation occurs).

Methylation is a biochemical process that helps to repair DNA at this intersection of the epigenome, which is where nutrients meet and communicate with your genes. We now know that DNA methylation plays a significant role in epigenetic gene regulation and the treatment of autoimmune disease.

The primary takeaway here is that it's possible to help control inflammation at the level of the epigenome via methylation by ensuring that we have the exact nutrients poised to silence inflammatory gene expression. That is, if the right nutrients are lined up, inflammatory gene switches get dimmed down and won't result in autoimmune reactions.

We also know that many patients with autoimmune conditions are genetically predisposed to methylation defects and need to consider supplementing with specific forms of folate, vitamin B6, and vitamin B12 to ensure proper methylation.

When you don't have the proper nutrition to support methylation, you may not be able to "dim down" your inflammatory gene switches effectively.

So how can you support methylation? You can start with a daily green smoothie and dark leafy greens, which are both good sources of the nutrients required for proper methylation. Some may need to consider specific methylation nutrients like methyl folate (5-MTHF), methyl B6 (P5P), and methyl B12. These specific forms of B vitamins are not only great for methylation but also help boost glutathione production and recycling in your body. However, please note that not everyone can utilize methyl forms of B vitamins and may do well with e.g. hydroxy B12, adenosyl B12, and/or cyano B12. A good way to find out which forms of B vitamins are most suitable for you would be to do Single Nucleotide Polymorphism (SNP) analysis starting with a 23andMe test.

2. Silence Nuclear Factor Kappa Beta

Nuclear Factor Kappa Beta (NFKB) is a DNA transcription factor that stimulates pro-inflammatory gene expression. To put it another way, when NFKB is activated, we feel inflamed.

NFKB can be activated by leaky gut, dysbiosis, SIBO, food sensitivities, stress, chemical exposures, and viruses. This in turn can lead to an increased expression of the pro-inflammatory genes that code for the production of inflammatory cytokines that make us feel inflamed.

By applying Functional Medicine, we can root out the trigger of this inflammatory response by eliminating poorly digested proteins, resolving dysbiosis, SIBO, battling infections, and healing your leaky gut. We can also modulate NFKB with botanicals like curcumin.

3. Increase Regulatory T-Cells and Self Tolerance

Probably, the most important thing you can do for an imbalanced immune system is to support regulatory T-cells (also known as TH3 cells). These cells keep all facets of the immune system in check by regulating the activity of TH1, TH2, and TH17. When the T-cells don't function properly, the immune system can tip out of balance and promote inflammation and autoimmunity.

When your immune system becomes dysregulated due to T-cell problems, you can suffer from self-tissue attack. This is the basic definition of "autoimmunity" and is also referred to as loss of self-tolerance. Increasing your regulatory T-cells is a way of restoring self-tolerance and balance to the immune system.

Pharmaceutical companies are spending billions of dollars to develop drugs that build up regulatory T-cells. Hopefully these products will be useful for treating autoimmunity in the future. There has also been some promising research on low-dose naltrexone (LDN) for helping to build up regulatory T-cells.

You can start decreasing inflammation now in a much more natural way. Start by getting on a Paleo autoimmune plan and by talking to a knowledgeable Functional Medicine health care practitioner to discuss your options for regulating the immune system and fighting inflammation.

THE IMPORTANCE OF HAPPINESS

It's often said that happiness is the key to life. Well, it's been shown that happiness can also play a factor in your well-being when it comes to autoimmune disease.

It's now recognized that regulatory T-cells are primed with receptors for vitamin D, glutathione, and endorphins. So, while the Paleo autoimmune diet is powerful in and of itself, it's only one part of a larger comprehensive protocol for halting autoimmune reactions.

The primary takeaway here is that happiness plays an important role in your overall health. And everyone needs to prioritize having more fun in life! Laughing more often, having a good time with friends, and even watching funny movies may give you the leverage you need to increase your regulatory T-cells and decrease your stress.

To put it in a scientific equation, TH3>TH17=Balanced Immune Function.

VITAMINS, FOOD AND SUPPLEMENTS FOR IMMUNE REGULATION

MICRONUTRITION SUPPORT

According to researcher Sarah Ballantyne Ph.D., patients with autoimmune conditions generally have deficiencies in vitamins A, B, C, D, E, K, zinc, copper, iron, magnesium, and selenium, as well as deficiencies of CoQ-10, Omega 3s, glycine, and fiber. Since these are all critical for proper immune cell function, one of the goals of the nutrient-dense Paleo autoimmune diet is to provide you with a good supply of these vitamins and minerals from the food you eat.

Since we now know that building regulatory T-cells is one of the most important things you can you for your immune system, let's look at the most significant vitamins and supplements for supporting regulatory T-cells:

- Vitamin D
- Fish oil, EPA/DHA
- Non-dairy probiotic strains
- Vitamin A
- Glutathione

VITAMIN D

Vitamin D is a cornerstone to good health. Research shows, however, that many people do not get enough of this important vitamin from sunlight and diet alone. In today's society, many people spend the bulk of their lives indoors, wear sunscreen when outside, and don't eat a vitamin D-rich diet.

More than 40 percent of the general population (and 60 percent of children) are estimated to be deficient in vitamin D. Factors such as obesity, aging, and living in a northern latitude have been found to increase the risk for vitamin D deficiency.

If you suffer from an autoimmune disease or other chronic illness, you can boost your level of vitamin D (Cholecalciferol) to support regulatory T-cell production and help you outpace and prevent disease. You can get vitamin D via supplements, though I recommend getting tested for vitamin D levels before going that route. You can also get vitamin D naturally from cod liver oil, herring, trout, salmon, halibut, mushrooms, beef liver, and sunshine.

FISH OIL, EPA/DHA

Omega 3 fatty acids also support regulatory T-cells. Besides supplementing with fish oil capsules, you can increase your intake of Omega 3 by including salmon, sardines, tuna, mackerel, and grass-fed meats in your diet.

PROBIOTICS

Probiotics help to replenish flora in your gut. Besides supplementing your diet with non-dairy probiotics, you can replenish good gut flora by making sure your diet includes foods like sauerkraut, coconut yogurt, kimchee, kombucha, and coconut kefir.

VITAMIN A

You can obtain vitamin A from liver, sweet potatoes, carrots, dark leafy greens, butternut squash, pumpkin, and cod liver oil.

GLUTATHIONE

Glutathione is the body's primary antioxidant. It's necessary for defending and repairing the gut lining. Although our body naturally makes and recycles glutathione, modern life can overwhelm our system and deplete us of this vital compound. When our glutathione level is low, our body is more vulnerable to disease and damage.

Glutathione's job is to protect the cells, whether it's from an autoimmune disease, sleep deprivation, or the toxic ingredients in scented detergents and fabric softeners. Healthy glutathione levels reduce your risk of developing chronic and autoimmune disease as well as food and chemical sensitivities.

Sulfur-rich foods such as garlic, onions, broccoli, kale, collards, cabbage, Brussels sprouts, leeks, chives, mustard greens, avocado, cauliflower, sweet potatoes and watercress can help boost glutathione. Epsom salt bathes are also recommended. Exercise also boosts glutathione, so make sure to get aerobic exercise daily (such as walking) and strength training two to three times a week. One of the most important ways to maintain your glutathione levels is to reduce stress on your body.

Glutathione as a supplement is not well absorbed by the digestive tract. Fortunately, many nutritional compounds act as building blocks to glutathione and can help raise and maintain its level inside and outside of cells. The nutrients shown below are some of best nutritional compounds for boosting glutathione (our primary antioxidant), which thereby supports regulatory T-cells and helps ensure a more balanced immune system:

- N-Acetyl Cysteine
- Alpha lipoic acid
- L-glutamine
- Milk Thistle
- Centella Asiatica
- Selenium
- Vitamin C
- Folate
- B6
- B12

These powerful botanicals, vitamins, and compounds all work by supporting regulatory T-cells. Glutathione can also be taken intravenously. You may also focus on the following food sources for optimal immune health.

Food sources of Vitamin B6: pork, mustard greens, cabbage, collard greens, leeks, garlic, tuna, cod, chard, calf's liver, turkey, salmon, cauliflower, kale, broccoli.

Food sources of B12: beef liver, clams, trout, salmon, lamb, halibut, shrimp and grass fed beef.

Food sources of Vitamin C: oranges, clementines, kiwi, guava, thyme, parsley, kale, mustard greens.

Food sources of Selenium: cod, shrimp, salmon, cod, tuna, button mushrooms.

Food sources of L-glutamine: beef, chicken, fish and bone broth.

Food sources of alpha lipoic acid: organ meats e.g heart, liver, kidney, broccoli and spinach

Glutathione is extremely important to your health. That's why it's imperative to have an awareness of how to prevent its depletion and ensure you do everything in your power to keep it at a high level.

STRATEGIES TO PREVENT GLUTATHIONE DEPLETION

Because glutathione is such an important factor in your health, I've included some strategies here for helping to boost glutathione levels.

- **Find out what your food intolerances are and remove those foods from your diet.** You can use the advanced Paleo autoimmune protocol, which is essentially an elimination diet, or a lab test, to help determine which foods are putting stress on your immune system and taxing your glutathione reserves.
- **Stick to the Paleo autoimmune dietary template.** Processed foods and fast foods contain chemical additives, genetic alterations, antibiotics, hormones, excess sugar, and other ingredients that deplete glutathione and put stress on your body.
- **Get enough sleep.** Sleep deprivation is very stressful to your body. If you have a sleeping problem, it's often secondary to something else.
- **Manage your autoimmune disease.** An autoimmune or chronic disease (such as Hashimoto's hypothyroidism, rheumatoid arthritis, or diabetes) keeps your immune system on overdrive and damages tissue, which depletes glutathione.

- **Reduce your exposure to toxins and pollutants.** Many common environmental chemicals are toxic to the body. They can be found in shampoos, body products, household cleaners, lawn-care products, and so on. We have enough to deal with in terms of pollutants in our air and water, minimize your exposure to these harmful substances in your home.
- **Minimize your exposure to EMFs.** Electromagnetic Fields (EMFs) are a source of "electrical pollution." Cell phones, computers, Wi-Fi, and other electronics put stress on the body.
- Avoid smoking, drinking, overtraining, and medications.

Any inflammation in the body puts an extra demand on glutathione and depletes it. On top of this, NFKB is activated, which causes us to become systemically inflamed and turns on inducible nitric oxide synthase (iNOS). This causes tissue damage and more inflammation along with putting a greater demand on glutathione.

SUPPORTING NITRIC OXIDE SYSTEM PATHWAYS

When NFKB is activated, the systemic inflammation turns on inducible nitric oxide synthase (iNOS), which causes tissue damage and more inflammation. You can use the following natural substances to help dampen this inflammation and facilitate tissue repair which then leads to decreased glutathione need.

- Huperzine A
- Vinpocetine
- Adenosine
- Alpha-Ketogluteric Acid
- L Acetylcarnitine

SUPPLEMENT AND HERB GUIDE

We now realize that certain herbs, botanicals, and supplements may be adversely "immune stimulating" for the autoimmune patient.

It's imperative, therefore, that you are aware of the potential adverse effects of using certain "immune stimulating" ingredients in supplements, such as maitake mushrooms and even lemon balm that's in many sleep supplements. You also need to look at the fillers included in many "whole food" supplements and medicines—many of them contain gluten.

Unfortunately, there are many well-meaning practitioners currently treating patients with autoimmune disease who lack the proper training in the immune-stimulating properties of botanicals and even in the foods they're recommending. Needless to say, it's extremely important for you to read labels carefully to make sure you're not inadvertently taking immune modulating, immune stimulating, or "immune boosting" herbs, botanicals or compounds such as Echinacea purpurea extract, astragalus, ashwaganda, beta glucans, chlorella, caffeine, coffee, goldenseal, grape seed extract, lycopene, licorice root (except DGL), Melissa officinalis (lemon balm), Maitake, pycnogenol, genistein, pine bark extract, panax ginseng, quercetin, Reishi, Shiitake, spirulina, and willow bark.

The chart in this section highlights the supplements that I've found to be most effective for the patients who I've treated for autoimmune conditions.

In general, I recommend Apex supplements, which have been formulated by Dr. Datis Kharrazian. Dr. Kharrazian is an excellent Functional Medicine instructor and the author of two informative books called *Why Do I Still Have Thyroid Symptoms When my Blood Tests are Normal?* and *Why Isn't My Brain Working?* These books are worth reading for anyone with concerns about autoimmune conditions.

I've also seen great results from some Metagenics products over the years. Metagenics was founded by Dr. Jeffrey Bland, a teacher and leader in the field of nutrition research for chronic disease management.

IMPORTANT NOTE: I've used some supplements by both of these manufacturers to successfully treat patients with autoimmunity. However, each patient is different. And certain supplements may not be appropriate for some patients suffering from autoimmune disease. In my practice, I monitor my patients closely, am aware of the condition of their immune system, and can appropriately recommend supplements specific to each case. It's always important to use these supplements with the guidance of a trained practitioner who understands your immune system imbalance, knows what's growing in your gut, has run the appropriate lab work, and who can help you understand clearly which supplements may be the most helpful for healing your autoimmune reactions.

The Autoimmune Paleo Breakthrough Supplement and Herb Guide

Regulatory T-cell Support			
Product	**Manufacturer**	**Product**	**Manufacturer**
• Omegagenics EPA/DHA	Metagenics	• AC glutathione	Apex Energetics
• Ultra Flora Plus DF	Metagenics	• Strengtia	Apex Energetics
• D3 5000	Metagenics	• Liqua-D	Apex Energetics
• Glutaclear	Metagenics		

General Vitamin Support	
Product	**Manufacturer**
• C Ultra Tabs	Metagenics
• Magnesium Glycinate	Metagenics

General GI Support			
Product	**Manufacturer**	**Product**	**Manufacturer**
• Metagest	Metagenics	• Super Digestzyme	Apex Energetics
• Metazyme	Metagenics	• HCL Prozyme	Apex Energetics
• Zinlori	Metagenics	• Gastro ULC	Apex Energetics

Methylation and Detoxification Support			
Product	**Manufacturer**	**Product**	**Manufacturer**
• Actifolate	Metagenics	• AC Glutathione	Apex Energetics
• Folapro	Metagenics		

Adrenal Support			
Product	**Manufacturer**	**Product**	**Manufacturer**
• Cortico B5, B6	Metagenics	• Corticozyme	Apex Energetics

Reduce Inflammation			
Product	**Manufacturer**	**Product**	**Manufacturer**
• Omegagenics EPA/DHA	Metagenics	• Nitric Balance	Apex Energetics
• Inflavonoid	Metagenics	• AC Glutathione	Apex Energetics

Brain Support			
Product	**Manufacturer**	**Product**	**Manufacturer**
• Omegagenics DHA 600	Metagenics	• Acetyl Ch	Apex Energetics
• St. John's Wort with Folate and B12	Metagenics	• Neuro Flam NT	Apex Energetics

For help designing a personalized Autoimmune Paleo Nutrition and Functional Medicine treatment program, please visit
www.paleobreakthrough.com

THE SHORT LIST OF SUPPLEMENTS FOR REVERSING AUTOIMMUNE REACTIONS

The supplements listed in this section are on my short list of botanicals that I recommend to my patients suffering from autoimmune disease. For actual product names, please see the supplement guide in the chart above.

REGULATORY T-CELL SUPPORT

EPA/DHA, Non-Dairy Probiotics, vitamin D (test first before supplementing), and by supporting glutathione with precursors (N-Acetyl Cysteine, Alpha Lipoic Acid, L-glutamine, Milk Thistle, Centella Asiatica, vitamin C, and Selenium).

IMPORTANT NOTE: *N-Acetyl Cysteine is not appropriate in the case of candida infection.*

REDUCE INFLAMMATION

Curcumin, EPA/DHA, Glutathione

SUPPORT DETOXIFICATION AND METHYLATION

Folate, B6, and B12 (check your SNP's first with a test such as 23andMe)

LEAKY GUT SUPPORT

L-Glutamine, zinc L-Carnosine, DGL, and probiotic foods.

GENERAL GI SUPPORT

Digestive enzymes, Ox Bile, and hydrochloric acid (always consult with a practitioner who is familiar with hydrochloric acid dosing before using hydrochloric acid tablets).

GENERAL VITAMIN SUPPORT

Magnesium glycinate, vitamin C.

FOR DYSBIOSIS, SIBO, PARASITES:

For SIBO specifically, if a starch free version of the Paleo autoimmune protocol isn't enough to resolve symptoms (i.e by removing SIBO caution foods), you may need to consider using antibiotics such as Xifaxin and/or botanical medicines.

IMPORTANT NOTE: While herbs are routinely used for gastrointestinal infections, many of the botanicals in this class for killing yeast, bacteria, and parasites are potential TH1 immune stimulants and are best used under the guidance of a knowledgeable practitioner who can help you to understand how to treat your immune system imbalance. Please don't use these supplements without the guidance of a trained practitioner who understands your immune system imbalance, knows what's growing in your gut, has run the appropriate lab work, and who can help you understand clearly which supplements may be the most helpful for healing your autoimmune reactions.

TRANSITIONING TO THE AUTOIMMUNE PROTOCOL FROM THE STANDARD AMERICAN DIET (THE FOUR-DAY TRANSITION)

If you're transitioning to the advanced Paleo autoimmune diet from the Standard American Diet (SAD), you may find the following transition guidelines to be helpful.

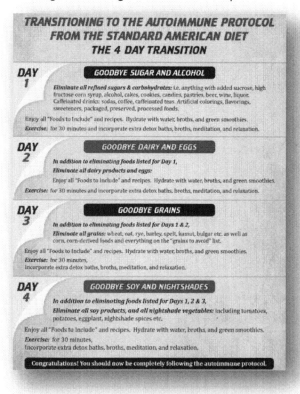

DETOX SUPPORT WHILE TRANSITIONING TO THE AUTOIMMUNE PROTOCOL

For anyone transitioning to the autoimmune Paleo template from the Standard American Diet, a grain-based gluten-free diet, or even a standard Paleo diet, you may benefit from the information in this section as your body adjusts to the autoimmune protocol.

DETOX SUPPORT
WHILE TRANSITIONING TO THE AUTOIMMUNE PROTOCOL

All those transitioning from either the standard American diet, a grain based gluten free diet, or even the standard Paleo diet, may benefit from this extra support as your body adjusts to the autoimmune protocol.

DETOX BATH RECIPE:

- 2 pounds of Epsom Salt plus
- 2 pounds of baking soda
- 10 drops of lavender essential oil

DETOX BROTH:

- 3 quarts of water
- 1 large chopped onion
- 2 sliced carrots
- 1 cup of daikon
- 1 cup of turnips and rutabaga cut into large cubes
- 2 cups of chopped greens: kale, parsley, beet greens, collard greens, chard, dandelion, cilantro or other greens
- 2 celery stalks
- ½ cup of cabbage
- 4 ½ inch slices of ginger
- 2 cloves of whole garlic
- Sea salt to taste

Add all the ingredients at once and place on low boil for 60 minutes. Cool and strain veggies out-discard them.

Makes approximately 8 cups. Store in fridge. Heat and drink 3-4 cups/day.

LIVER SUPPORT:

Try a shot of olive oil & lemon juice (one tablespoon of each mixed with 4 oz. of water).

FOODS FOR LIVER DETOX:

Protein, kale, broccoli, cabbage, cauliflower, Brussels sprouts, beets.

SUPPLEMENTS FOR LIVER DETOX:

Milk thistle, Glutathione and it's precursors, L- Glutamine, L- Glycine and L-Cysteine (NAC).

RAW APPLE CIDER VINEGAR:

1 tablespoon diluted with 1 tablespoon in water helps your stomach produce hydrochloric acid, and aid digestion of proteins.

FOR BODY ACHES, HEADACHES AND CONSTIPATION:

- 800 mg Magnesium glycinate

EASY EXERCISE:

30 minute walk per day.

STRESS REDUCTION

Reducing stress is an important factor in improving immune system balance and overall health. I've found that along with acupuncture and massage therapy; exercise (in my case swimming), yoga, and meditation have helped provide me with a greater awareness of my own capacity to regulate my nervous system and immune system. Mindful breathing, in particular, in yoga and other activities helps to balance the nervous system.

Visualization can also be a helpful practice. In the Chinese Medical Qi Gong therapy, for instance, patients are instructed to visualize what it's like to be healed as the practitioner does the same. Using visualization to imagine being healed can be a powerful technique that is well worth cultivating.

I also recommend finding a good yoga studio, an acupuncturist, a meditation class, and doing everything else in your power to prevent stress from entering your body. Daily Epsom salt baths are another effective way of helping to manage stress.

THE 30-DAY ELIMINATION CHALLENGE

GETTING STARTED

The advanced Paleo autoimmune plan is designed to rapidly reduce inflammation and heal intestinal permeability via specific dietary interventions. To calm down your immune/inflammatory response and allow the gut to heal, you'll need to remove the major offending foods, including eggs, grains, alcohol, nightshades, nuts, seeds, legumes, and dairy for at least 30 days. This is referred to as the elimination phase of the diet.

Once you start this plan, your dietary emphasis will be on whole, organic, and nutrient-dense foods, which all contribute to optimal digestion and immune function. You'll be eating many anti-inflammatory and antioxidant rich fruit and veggies. The veggies and protein you'll be eating will boost your minerals and amino acids, which will help to stabilize your blood sugar and strengthen your adrenals. You are encouraged to eat 3 meals/day without skipping any meals. Besides not skipping meals, eating a small amount of protein at each meal is a great way to you're your blood sugar balanced. You'll also reduce intestinal inflammation and get a lot of nutrients necessary for healthy intestinal micro-flora through probiotic and cultured foods. Add to that lots of water and herbal teas and you'll be off to a great start.

In general, you're encouraged to eat pastured, grass-fed meat, wild fish, plenty of vegetables, healthy fats (from salmon, mackerel, coconut, avocado, and olives), and fermented foods (such as sauerkraut, kombucha, coconut kefir, and yogurt), along with plenty of water, green smoothies, and non-caffeinated herbal teas.

Sarah Ballantyne, Ph.D. (aka The Paleo Mom) recommends focusing on good quality (pastured, grass fed) organ meat, and glycine-rich bone broth at least five times per week. Try to get at least three servings per week of fish and/or shellfish along with many veggies and sea vegetables (e.g., seaweed). Keep your daily fructose intake to less than 20g/day.

You're encouraged to eat the foods on the "Foods to Include" list included in the book, with the caveat that you should avoid any foods that you suspect are problematic and do not agree with your constitution. As a general rule, avoid thinking about what you can't eat, and instead focus on all the foods you CAN eat!

After 30 days on this plan you should notice significant health benefits, including decreased autoimmune reactions, decreased inflammation, increased mental clarity, improved digestion, and better mood and energy. Each person will react differently on this diet, and some patients take longer to see results. Some who go on this diet will need to continue strictly on this plan for one year or longer before introducing any potential food triggers back into their diet.

If you don't improve while on this advanced Paleo autoimmune Paleo protocol, you'll have to do further investigation and consider other aspects that might be driving your autoimmune reactions. For instance, some patients will need to check for SIBO, dysbiosis and/or FODMAP intolerance, cross-reactive proteins, hidden infections, hormonal imbalances, and chemical exposures.

If autoimmune symptoms come back after you go off the Paleo autoimmune protocol, you can always return to the diet to decrease your inflammatory response. Always check with your health care practitioner if you have a flare-up of symptoms.

The Paleo autoimmune plan guidelines are summarized in the following chart.

AUTOIMMUNE PROTOCOL GUIDELINES

- Eat fermented foods like sauerkraut, coconut kefir, and yogurt.
- Drink 8 glasses of water including veggie or bone broth daily.
- Eat organic, pastured, grass fed animal protein and wild fish.
- Eat low glycemic fruits and non-starchy vegetables.
- No genetically modified organism (GMO) foods.
- Eat carbohydrates from fruits and vegetables.
- Eat fat from avocados, coconut, and olive oil.
- Get a few servings of organ meat per week.
- Meditate for at least 5 minutes per day.
- Eat fiber from fruits and vegetables.
- Eat Superfoods on a daily basis.
- Drink green smoothies daily.
- Get 7-9 hours of sleep.
- No dairy products.
- No fruit juices.
- No eggs.
- No grains at all.
- No refined sugars.
- No skipping meals.
- No wine or alcohol.
- No processed foods.
- No nightshade vegetables.
- No smoked or salted foods.
- No cereals or grain like seeds.
- No nuts, seeds or seed based spices.
- Get 5 servings of bone broth per week.
- Get 3 servings of omega 3 rich fish per week.
- Exercise every day, preferably for 30 minutes.
- No ibuprofen, aspirin, acetaminophen, naproxen.
- Take daily detox baths with Epsom salts, and baking soda.
- No legumes (e.g. peanuts, beans, lentils, peas, and soybeans).
- Consider digestive enzymes, hydrochloric acid, and apple cider vinegar to facilitate digestion.

A word about caution foods on the autoimmune protocol food lists:

Generally speaking, these foods are either immunogenic, hard to digest, likely to feed gut bacterial overgrowths, dysbiosis, and/or contribute to blood sugar imbalance. If your gut immunity is strong (no overgrowths, no dysbiosis, no food reactions, healthy gut lining), and your blood sugar is balanced, these items may be tolerated in moderation.

FOODS TO INCLUDE
AND ELIMINATE

This section includes a list of foods to include, as well as foods to eliminate from your diet. As mentioned in the previous chapter, be sure to focus on all the foods you CAN eat instead of lamenting over items you can no longer have! And, remember, the bottom line is that you're setting out on this dietary adventure in order to improve your health.

FOODS TO INCLUDE

FRUITS

Apples, apricots, Asian pears, bananas, blueberries, blackberry, boysenberry, cherries, clementines, cranberry, figs, guava, grapes, grapefruit, kiwi, lemons, limes, marionberry, mango, melons, nectarine, oranges, papaya, peaches, pears, persimmons, plums, pluots, plantains, pomegranate, raspberry, strawberry, tangerine, and watermelon.

VEGETABLES

Asparagus, arugula, artichoke, avocado, artichoke hearts, Brussels sprouts, basil, beet, beet greens, broccoli, broccoli rabe, burdock, bok choy, cabbage, carrots, cauliflower, celery, celeriac, chard, chicory, collards, chard, cucumber, daikon radish, dandelion greens, fennel root, green cabbage, green beans, jicama, Jerusalem artichoke, kale, kohlrabi, leeks, lettuce, mustard, Napa cabbage, nettles, okra, onions, purslane, red cabbage, radish, shallot, scallion, snap peas, spinach, summer squash, turnips, water chestnuts, watercress, and zucchini.

DENSE CARBS

Acorn squash, beets, butternut squash, plantain and lotus root, sweet potato, taro, and yams.

FUNGI

Button mushrooms, chanterelle, crimini, portabella, puffball, oyster, etc.

WILD FISH

Cod, flounder, herring, halibut, hake, mackerel, oysters, red snapper, salmon, shellfish, tuna, sardines, skate, trout, etc.

MEAT

Beef, buffalo, bison, chicken, Cornish game hen, duck, emu, goose, goat, organic sliced meats (gluten and sugar free), pasture-raised lamb, pork, ostrich, sausage (without fillers or nightshade spices), quail, squab, turkey, venison, uncured nitrate/nitrite-free deli meats, and bacon from grass-fed/pastured beef/pork.

OFFAL

Bone broth, liver, kidney, and heart.

MILK AND YOGURT

Coconut milk and unsweetened coconut yogurt.

FATS AND OILS

Coconut oil, extra virgin olive oil, flaxseed, hazelnut oil, sesame, red palm oil, walnut, animal fat, avocado oil, duck fat, and tallow.

CAUTION: Some patients may be sensitive to the following nut- and seed-based oils: Flaxseed oil, hazelnut oil, macadamia nut oil, sesame oil, and walnut oil.

COCONUT

Coconut oil, coconut butter, coconut milk, coconut cream, coconut aminos, coconut kefir, unsweetened coconut yogurt, and unsweetened coconut flakes.

BEVERAGES

Broths, coconut kefir, freshly-made veggie juice, filtered or distilled water, green smoothies, herbal tea, kombucha, kefir water, and mineral water.

TEAS

Herbal teas: peppermint, ginger, lemongrass, spearmint, chamomile, rooibos, lavender, cinnamon, and milk thistle.

In Moderation: Black and Green Tea

FERMENTED FOODS

Beet kvass, carrots, cucumbers, green papaya, kombucha, kimchee, kefir water, lacto-fermented vegetables and fruits such as fermented beets, pickles, pickled ginger, pickled unsweetened coconut yogurt, unsweetened coconut kefir (without corn- or rice-based thickening agents), pickles fermented with salt, and sauerkraut.

CONDIMENTS

Apple cider vinegar, Balsamic vinegar, coconut vinegar, Red Boat fish sauce, coconut aminos, and ume plum vinegar.

HERBS AND SPICES

Bay leaves, basil, chives, chamomile, chervil, cinnamon, cloves, cilantro, dill, garlic, ginger, horseradish, lemongrass, marjoram, mace, oregano, parsley, peppermint, rosemary, sage, sea, salt, spearmint, saffron, sea salt, shallots, turmeric, thyme, and tarragon.

CAUTION: Some patients may be sensitive to the following seed-based spices: Allspice, black pepper, cardamom, white, green, and pink peppercorns, juniper, star anise, and vanilla bean.

SUGAR SUBSTITUTES

Cinnamon, mint, and ginger.

CAUTION: Use the following items in moderation. Honey, *maple syrup, molasses, unrefined cane sugar, and date sugar.*

CAUTION FOODS TO INCLUDE IN MODERATION

A WORD ABOUT CAUTION FOODS

Generally speaking, these foods are either immunogenic, hard to digest, likely to feed gut bacterial overgrowths, dysbiosis, and/or contribute to blood sugar imbalance. These items may be tolerated in moderation If your gut immunity is strong (i.e., no overgrowths, no dysbiosis, no food reactions, and a healthy gut lining) and your blood sugar is balanced.

SWEETENERS

Honey, maple syrup, molasses, unrefined cane sugar, and date sugar should be used in moderation and not at all if you have dysbiosis and/or SIBO or fructose intolerance.

SPICES

Allspice, black pepper, cardamom, green and pink peppercorns, juniper, star anise, and vanilla bean may be irritating to a leaky gut.

NUT- AND SEED-BASED OILS

Flaxseed oil, hazelnut oil, sesame oil, walnut oil, and macadamia nut oil may be irritating to a leaky gut.

HIGH-GLYCEMIC FRUITS

Grapes, watermelon, mango, pineapple, dried fruits, and dehydrated fruits may feed dybiosis and dysregulate blood sugar. In general, it is recommended to keep your fructose consumption to below 20g per day (this can be 2-5 pieces per day, depending on the fruit). These fruits are fine in moderation IF you have a healthy gut without any overgrowths of SIBO or dysbiosis, stable blood sugar, and can tolerate fructose.

FOODS TO ELIMINATE

VEGGIES

Avoid all nightshade vegetables. This includes potatoes (but not sweet potatoes), all tomatoes, red and green peppers, chili peppers, eggplants, tomatillos, sweet bell peppers, jalapenos, cayenne, peppers (Habanero, Anaheim, Serrano, etc.) Avoid chili peppers in dried powders such as paprika, chili powder, curry powder, chili pepper flakes, hot sauces, Tabasco sauces, salsas, goji berries, and ashwaganda.

FRUIT

Avoid canned fruits.

PROCESSED AND CANNED MEATS

Bacon (unless gluten, dairy, and preservative free), deli meats, smoked/dried/salted meat and fish. Sausages and deli meats with seed-based or nightshade spices.

FISH

Whale, shark, and swordfish. Farmed tilapia and catfish should be eaten in moderation.

NUTS AND SEEDS

Avoid all nuts and seeds, including almonds, Brazil nuts, coffee, cocoa, cashews, chestnuts, hazelnuts, macadamias, pine nuts, pistachios, pumpkin, pecans, walnuts, and sunflower.

SEEDS AND SEED-BASED SPICES

Anise, annatto, black cumin, celery, coriander, canola, caraway, chia, dill, fennel, fenugreek, mustard, nutmeg, poppy, and sesame.

DAIRY

Butter, cow and other animal (goat/sheep) milks, cheese, cottage cheese, cream, frozen desserts, ghee, ice-cream, mayonnaise, non-dairy creamers, soy milk, whey, and yogurt.

FATS AND OIL

Avoid any processed hydrogenated oils, butter, margarine, mayonnaise, peanut oil, and shortening.

BEANS AND LEGUMES

Avoid all beans, black beans, black-eyed peas, cashews, chickpeas, kidney beans, lima beans, lentils, fava, miso, peas, peanuts/peanut butter, soybean, and soy products.

FUNGI

Avoid medicinal mushrooms (e.g., Shiitake, Maitake, and Reishi mushrooms).

SOY

Soymilk, soy sauce, tofu, tempeh, soy protein, and edamame.

BEVERAGES

All caffeinated beverages, alcoholic beverages, coffee, fruit juice, and soda.

CONDIMENTS

BBQ sauce, baker's and brewer's yeast, chutneys, ketchup, relish, soy sauce, and other condiments.

SWEETENERS

Avoid white and brown sugar, agave, brown rice syrup, corn syrup, Equal, fruit sweeteners, high-fructose corn syrup, maple syrup, NutraSweet, Splenda, stevia, Truvia, Xylitol, and raw green stevia.

GRAINS

Amaranth, barley, buckwheat, corn (including cornmeal and popcorn), cracked wheat and wheat berries, durum and other forms such as bulgur, emmer, farro, einkorn, millet, oats, oatmeal, quinoa, rice, rye, sorghum, teff, triticale, and wheat (including varieties such as spelt and kamut).

GRAIN PRODUCTS

Breads, cakes, corn tortillas, chips, crackers, cookies, cake, doughnuts, flat bread, muffins, noodles, pasta, pizza, pita, pancakes, rolls, starch, syrup, tortillas, and waffles.

GRAIN LIKE SUBSTANCES AND PSEUDO CEREALS

Amaranth, buckwheat, cattail, chia, cockscomb, goosefoot, pitseed, quinoa, kañiwa, and wattleseed (also known as acacia seed).

GLUTEN-CONTAINING FOODS

BBQ sauce, binders, bouillon, brewer's yeast, cold cuts, condiments, emulsifiers, fillers, gum, hot dogs, hydrolyzed plant and vegetable protein, ketchup, soy sauce, lunch meats, malt, malt flavoring, malt vinegar, matzo, modified food starch, monosodium glutamate, non-dairy creamer, processed salad dressings, seitan, stabilizers, teriyaki sauce, and textured vegetable protein.

LEGUMES

Beans, including peas, lentils, soy, and peanuts.

LECTINS

Avoid nuts, beans, eggplant, potatoes, tomato, peppers, peanut oil, peanut butter, soy, soy oil, etc.

DAIRY

All dairy products, including milk, cream, and cheese from cows, goats, sheep, etc.

EGGS

Avoid eggs and foods that contain eggs (e.g., mayonnaise).

ALCOHOL

Avoid all alcohol.

PROCESSED FOOD

Cured meats, canned foods, pre-mixed seasonings and sauces, mayonnaise, mustard, and sugar.

SUGARS

Avoid agave, brown rice syrup, coconut sugar, palm sugar, corn syrup, Equal, fruit sweeteners, high-fructose corn syrup, NutraSweet, raw green stevia, Splenda, stevia, Truvia, white or brown sugar, and Xylitol.

SEED-BASED SPICES

Anise, annatto, black cumin, celery, cacao, coriander, cumin, dill, fennel, fenugreek, mustard, nutmeg, poppy, and sesame.

BERRY- AND FRUIT-BASED SPICES

Allspice, black pepper, cardamom, green and pink peppercorns, juniper, star anise, and vanilla bean.

COFFEE

Remove coffee for 30 days and proceed with caution upon reintroducing it to your diet.

IMMUNE STIMULANTS

Echinacea purpurea extract, astragalus, ashwaganda, beta glucans, chlorella, caffeine, coffee, goldenseal, grape seed extract, lycopene, licorice root (except DGL), Melissa officinalis (lemon balm), Maitake, pycnogenol, genistein, pine bark extract, panax ginseng, quercetin, Reishi, Shiitake, spirulina, and willow bark.

CONGRATULATIONS ON COMPLETING THE 30+ DAY ELIMINATION PHASE: NOW LET'S TROUBLESHOOT

The following foods are included in the autoimmune protocol; however, they may still be problematic for some patients. If you're experiencing little to no improvement after thirty days, you may want to experiment further by eliminating other foods listed below.

FODMAPS AND FODMAP INTOLERANCE

FODMAPS describe the carbohydrates found in many common foods. FODMAP stands for Fermentable Oligo-, Di- and Mono-saccharides, and Polyols (sugar alcohols).

FODMAP intolerance can tip you off to the possibility of having enzyme deficiencies and/or having small intestine bacterial overgrowth. When poorly digested, the carbs from FODMAPs will feed bad bacteria (see SIBO below), which will in turn produce methane and hydrogen gas that can cause the bloating, cramping, burping, gas, diarrhea, and other bowel problems that are generally diagnosed as IBS.

Bacterial overgrowths that remain untreated may contribute to leaky gut and the inflammatory/immune response. FODMAP intolerance can indicate enzyme deficiencies, GLUT5 insufficiency, or the possibility of having small intestine bacterial overgrowth and/or dysbiosis, which may require further testing and follow up with a qualified health care professional.

If you have IBS symptoms and are not improving on the strict elimination phase of the Paleo autoimmune diet, the best way to check for FODMAP sensitivity would be to remove high-fructose fruits and other FODMAP foods for at least 30 days and then reintroduce them. You can also check for SIBO if there's still no change. If you want to reintroduce these foods to your diet, make sure you've resolved the root cause of your FODMAP intolerance to avoid symptoms.

FRUIT INTAKE FOR FODMAP INTOLERANCE

If you have a FODMAP intolerance, it is recommended to avoid high-fructose fruits (including dried fruits, cherries, apples, and pears). In addition, it is suggested to keep other fruit servings to below 20g of fructose/day.

FODMAPS IN THE PALEO PROTOCOL

Apples, artichokes, apricots, asparagus, avocado, beet root, blackberries, broccoli, Brussels sprouts, butternut squash, cabbage, cauliflower, celery, coconut flour, coconut milk, coconut cream, coconut butter, cherries, dried coconut, dried fruits, fennel bulb, garlic, grapes, honey, leeks, mushrooms, nectarines, okra, onions, pears, plum, persimmon, peaches, pluots, pumpkin, radicchio, and sauerkraut.

SIBO CAUTION FOODS IN THE PALEO PROTOCOL

Parsnips, yams, jicama, kohlrabi, okra, sweet potato, taro, plantain, Jerusalem artichoke, parsnips, lotus root, cassava root, manioc, tapioca, and yucca.

OTHER SUSPECT FOODS: THE NEXT FRONTIER

After giving your body some time to adjust to the autoimmune diet, you may notice much less inflammation and better immune function. Some patients may still need to explore other food sensitivities and other underlying triggers of poor digestion.

It's not suggested to go off high-salicylate, high-histamine, and high-oxalate foods in the elimination phase. However, if you're still experiencing symptoms after 30 days, you may want to add these categories of foods to your plan.

SALICYLATE SENSITIVITY

Salicylate sensitivity has the potential to create more inflammation in the body and has been linked to IBS, Crohn's disease, and Colitis. High-salicylate foods have also been linked to the following symptoms: itchy skin, hives or rashes, stomach pain, nausea and/or diarrhea, asthma, other breathing difficulties such as persistent cough, headaches, swelling of the hands and feet, tissue swelling of the eyelids, face, and/or lips (angioedema), changes in skin color, fatigue, sore, itchy, puffy or burning eyes, nasal congestion or sinusitis, memory loss and poor concentration (linked to ADHD), ringing in the ears, depression, and anxiety.

HIGH-SALICYLATE FOODS IN THE PROTOCOL

Berries, apricot, avocado, blackberry, cherries, plum/prune, green olives, endive, gherkin, radish, tangelo, tangerine, water chestnut, coconut oil, olive oil, all dried fruits, honey, date, grape, guava, orange, and pineapple.

HISTAMINE INTOLERANCE

Patients who have salicylate intolerance may also have histamine intolerance. Like FODMAP intolerance, histamine intolerance may tip you off to SIBO and/or dysbiotic bacteria and/or enzyme deficiencies.

In the case of bacterial overgrowth, the bacteria secrete histamine, and the enzyme system that breaks down histamine gets overwhelmed and results in allergic symptoms similar to salicylate intolerance (including nasal congestion, rashes, abdominal cramping, nausea, asthma, runny nose, itchy skin, watery eyes, hives, fatigue, headaches, irritability, heartburn, and angioedema). Many foods that are high in salicylates are also high in histamines.

HIGH-HISTAMINE FOODS

Bacon, berries, cloves, cinnamon, dried fruit, dry cured sausages, fermented ham, fermented cured meats, fermented sausages, grapefruit, kombucha, lemons, lime, leftover meat, mackerel, oranges, sauerkraut, shellfish, sauerkraut, sardines, spinach, vinegar, vinegar pickles, anchovy and anchovy paste, banana, fish sauce, fish paste, grape, pork, shrimp paste, strawberry, tuna, and tangerine.

HIGH-OXALATE FOODS

Foods that are high in oxalates can contribute to pain and inflammation.

HIGH-OXALATE FOODS IN THE PROTOCOL

Sweet potatoes, endive, asparagus, Brussels sprouts, cucumbers, celery and beets, chard, and beet greens.

The following high-oxalate foods are not in the Paleo autoimmune protocol, so you may want to consider them keeping them out of your diet altogether, or at least until you're condition improves: almonds, walnuts, cashews, pecans, sunflower, sesame, peanut, pinto beans, black beans, soy beans, rye, millet, oats, corn, potatoes, tea, coffee, and beer.

REINTRODUCTION OF FOODS

When reintroducing a food to your diet, do so one food at a time, then wait 72 hours to see if you have any reactions (e.g., headache, joint ache, skin rash, decreased mental clarity, etc.). Be sure to wait until the symptom subsides before reintroducing the next food.

WHAT CAN I EAT FIRST?

According to Sarah Ballantyne, Ph.D., who's also known as The Paleo Mom, try to reintroduce foods that are the least likely to be problematic, such as egg yolk, non-nightshade seed-based spices and starchy vegetables, seeds (except sesame), nuts, grass-fed butter, and alcohol.

You can then introduce foods that may be moderate triggers, including paprika, sweet peppers, eggplant, coffee, cocoa, chocolate, sesame seeds, cassava, yucca, manioc, yeast, grass fed raw cream and fermented grass-fed dairy. You should reintroduce goat milk dairy before cow milk dairy, since it seems like most patients can tolerate goat dairy better than cow dairy.

The worst offenders should be reintroduced last. These would include egg whites, chili peppers, NSAIDS, and tomatoes (which may actually be best avoided forever).

CROSS-REACTIVE PROTEINS

If you have gluten intolerance, as most people with autoimmune conditions do, proceed with caution if EVER reintroducing the following proteins: dairy proteins (casein, casomorphin, butyrophilin, and whey), oats, brewer/baker's yeast, instant coffee, sorghum, millet, corn, rice, and potato. These foods may cause the same antibody/inflammatory reaction as gluten.

IMPORTANT NOTE: Since the reintroduction of foods may cause pronounced reactions, you should always inform your health care practitioner when you're thinking about reintroducing foods.

TROUBLESHOOTING THE AUTOIMMUNE PROTOCOL

Most patients feel much less inflamed when they go on the Paleo autoimmune protocol. They tend to have better digestion and energy along with markedly decreased autoimmune reactions. Other patients, though, may still experience digestive distress from certain foods. Rather than throwing in the towel and dismissing the protocol altogether, you're encouraged to view your symptoms as a clinical clue for further investigation. Follow the clues until you find the answer to your autoimmune condition.

If you continue having symptoms after sticking to the Paleo autoimmune plan, you may need to investigate the following:

- Is it time to do blood work to check for anemia, blood sugar issues, or hidden infections?
- Is it time to consider a comprehensive digestive analysis?
- Do you have SIBO that needs to be treated?
- Do you have leaky gut that needs specific therapeutic supplementation?
- Should you consider avoiding FODMAPs, high-histamine, high-salicylate, and high-oxalate foods?

- Should you consider adding supplements to aid in decreasing your inflammation and hacking gene expression on a daily basis?
- Do you need to balance blood sugar, aid in supporting your adrenal health, and/or aid in detoxification/methylation?
- Is it time to take sleep hygiene more seriously and start protecting your circadian rhythms?

You can refer to the following reference chart to consider your next step(s) in combatting your autoimmune disease. As mentioned throughout this book, you should also work with a knowledgeable health care practitioner (if you aren't already) to get to the bottom of what's happening with your immune system.

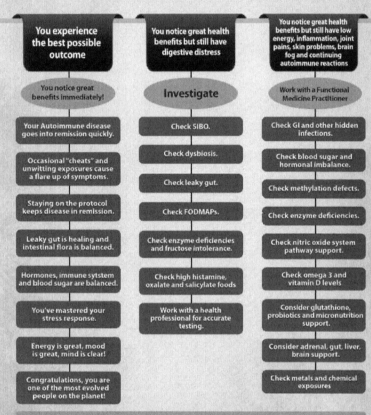

WORKING WITH A PRACTITIONER WHO UNDERSTANDS FUNCTIONAL MEDICINE, PALEO PRINCIPLES, AND AUTOIMMUNE DISEASE

Work with a Functional Medicine practitioner who can order relevant testing for auto-antibodies, infections, blood sugar and hormonal imbalances, dysbiosis, adrenal stress, liver detoxification, intestinal permeability, gluten sensitivity, cross-reactive proteins, SIBO, and lactose and fructose malabsorption.

Once the factors contributing to your autoimmune reactions have been identified, your Functional Medicine practitioner will treat your condition by using a variety of science-backed, non-pharmaceutical approaches. These approaches include:

- Adjusting your diet toward a more appropriate Paleo autoimmune template.
- Changing your lifestyle to improve health. Suggested changes could include eating breakfast, proper sleep habits, physical activity, stress reduction, etc.
- Suggesting botanicals or nutritional compounds to improve your health.
- Using lab-based testing to identify and recommend other natural medicine approaches.

Your Functional Medicine practitioner will work with you to uncover the root cause of your inflammation. You might get frustrated at times by what seems like a lack of progress in treating your condition, but stick with it. With patience and perseverance, and with the guidance of a knowledgeable practitioner, you can ultimately turn your health around.

CHECKLIST FOR TREATING AUTOIMMUNE DISEASE

When working with your Functional Medicine practitioner, here's a quick checklist of things to consider when treating autoimmune disease.

- Support regulatory T-cells with the following: EPA/DHA, probiotics, and vitamin D. And also by supporting glutathione with N-Acetyl Cysteine, Alpha lipoic acid, L-glutamine, Milk Thistle, Centella Asiatica, and Selenium.
- Clear your body of dysbiosis and SIBO with antimicrobial, anti-parasitic, and/or anti-fungal botanicals and/or pharmaceuticals.
- Support the integrity of your gut lining with L-Glutamine, zinc, DGL, and probiotic foods.
- Add digestive enzymes and hydrochloric acid for gas and bloating.
- Reduce inflammation with curcumin, EPA/DHA, and glutathione.
- Support detoxification and methylation if needed with folate, B6, and B12.
- Manage your stress.
- Cool your inflammation.
- Eat more plants.
- Check for FODMAPs.
- Check for hidden infections.
- Eat nutrient-dense protein.

- Maintain a healthy gut.
- Exercise for 30 minutes/day.
- Get more sleep->ideally 7-9 hours/night
- Stabilize your blood sugar.
- Support your adrenals
- Balance your hormones.
- Meditate.

Lastly, have fun! As discussed previously, adding more fun and laughter to your life can play a critical role in improving your overall health. Of course, it's not fun to suffer from autoimmune disease, but you can get enjoyment out of learning about your body and trying all sorts of new recipes as you move forward on the path to improving your autoimmune condition.

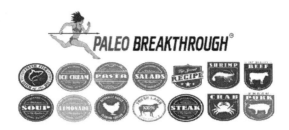

DELICIOUS AIP FRIENDLY RECIPES

TRI-TIP STEAK AND ASPARAGUS

Serv ings: 3

- Tri-tip steak (1 pound)
- 1 head of asparagus
- olive oil
- sea salt
- 2 sprigs of fresh rosemary

Coat everything with olive oil, chopped rosemary, and salt. Grill to perfection.

BONE BROTH

- 4 quarts water
- 2 lbs beef bones (or oxtail)
- 6 garlic cloves
- 3 ribs of celery
- 1 onion chopped
- 2 tablespoon apple cider vinegar
- 1 teaspoon sea salt

Place all ingredients in a pot and bring the stock to a boil, then reduce the heat to low and allow the stock to cook for 8 hours. Allow the stock to cool then strain to discard bones, etc. Store the stock in the fridge and use within a few days.

BEEF STEW

Servings: 4-6

- Grass-fed beef brisket 3 lbs.
- 10 garlic cloves, peeled
- salt to taste
- 1 bay leaf
- 1 ½ cups beef broth
- 8 cups of veggies, leeks, carrots, celery, and onions.

Cut slits into beef and add peeled garlic cloves in each. Sprinkle salt on beef. Chop up your veggies and add all ingredients to the slow cooker. Set on high for 4 hours or low   for   8   hours.

VEGGIE STEW

- 1 and ½ cups water, divided
- 4 cups sliced onion
- 2 cups thinly sliced leek
- 1 1/2 cups (1/2-inch-thick) sliced carrots
- 3 cups (1-inch) cubed daikon (about 1 pound)
- 1 bay leaf
- 4 cups (1-inch) cubed zucchini (about 1 1/2 pounds)
- 1/2 teaspoon ground cinnamon
- dash of saffron
- 4 garlic cloves, minced
- 6 cups chopped Swiss chard (about 12 ounces)
- 1/2 cup chopped cilantro
- 2 1/2 teaspoons salt, divided
- 2 tablespoons fresh lemon juice

Add all ingredients to a crock-pot or slow cooker. Cook on high heat for 2-3 hours.

PORK TENDERLOIN

Servings: 6

- 8 garlic cloves, coarsely chopped
- 1 tablespoon fresh oregano, finely chopped
- 1 tablespoon fresh thyme, finely chopped
- 1 tablespoon fresh rosemary, finely chopped
- 1 teaspoon salt
- 1/4 cup balsamic vinegar
- 1/2 cup olive oil
- 2 one pound pork tenderloins

Marinade pork for up to 24 hrs in ingredients above. Grill to perfection.

GARLIC ROSEMARY SALMON

Servings: 2

- 2 salmon fillets
- 5 cloves garlic, crushed
- olive oil (enough to coat the salmon)
- dried rosemary to taste
- the juice from 1 lemon

Mix garlic with dill, olive oil, lemon, and coat the salmon. Grill to perfection.

GINGER SALMON AND BROCCOLI

Servings: 4

- 1 head broccoli, cut into florets
- 2 TBSP coconut oil
- Sea salt
- 1 pound salmon
- squeeze of lemon
- ¼ bunch fresh cilantro
- 1 TBSP ginger, chopped
- 2 TBSP coconut aminos

Cover salmon with coconut oil, cilantro, ginger, coconut aminos, and a squeeze of lemon. Grill pan to perfection and serve with steamed broccoli.

BAKED TILAPIA WITH LEMON AND FRESH HERBS

Servings: 4

- 1 shallot, finely chopped
- 4 tilapia fillets
- 4 teaspoons olive oil
- sea salt
- 1 teaspoon finely chopped fresh thyme leaves
- ½ TBSP chopped parsley
- ½ TBSP fresh cilantro
- 1 teaspoon salt
- finely grated zest of 2 lemons

Mix herbs and seasonings with olive oil. Add Lemon zest and spread half of seasoning over fish. Place fish in broiler pan lined with parchment paper. Broil in pre-heated broiler for 3 minutes. Turn fish, applying remaining seasoning and broil for 3-5 minutes.

CROCK POT CHICKEN

Servings: 6

- 2.5 lbs. boneless, skinless chicken thighs
- 3 parsnips
- 3 carrots
- 4 celery stalks
- 1 red onion
- 10-12 whole garlic cloves
- 1/4 cup coconut oil
- 1 cup chicken broth
- 1 TSP fresh sage
- Sea salt to taste

Add everything to your crockpot and let cook on high for 4 hours.

GRILL PAN CHICKEN COLLARD WRAP

Servings: 2

- 6 collard leaves, cut lengthwise into two large pieces (stems removed)
- carrot, cucumber, celery, cut into sticks
- handful of cilantro, whole or chopped
- avocado, sliced into wedges
- 2 organic chicken breasts coated with olive oil thyme and sea salt

Grill chicken, cut into slices and make a wrap with crunchy veggies inside the collard greens.

ROAST CHICKEN

Servings: 2-4

- 1 whole chicken, 6 lbs.
- 1 lime, juiced
- 1/2 bunch cilantro
- 3 green onions, chopped
- 6 cloves garlic, peeled
- 1/4 cup olive oil
- 1 TBSP coconut oil
- salt

Chop and mix ingredients, rub chicken. Bake at 400 degrees for 45 minutes.

PALEO PAILLARD

Servings: 5

- 5 chicken breasts
- salt to taste
- 1/2 cup coconut flour
- 3 TBSP olive or coconut oil
- 1 cup chicken broth
- 3 TBSP capers, drained and rinsed
- 4 sprigs fresh thyme

Coat chicken with olive oil and salt, and then dip in coconut flour. Transfer chicken in a single layer to hot skillet and cook chicken cutlets 3 to 4 minutes on each side with capers and thyme. Add broth and cook for 15 minutes.

SUPERSONIC SALAD

- 1 cup butter lettuce
- 1 cup spinach
- 1/2 cup dino kale (shredded)
- 1/4 cup parsley
- 1/8 cup fresh basil
- 1/8 cup carrots (diced or shredded)
- 1/8 cup celery (diced)

MEDITERRANIAN SALAD

Ingredients:

- 2 cups red or green-leafed lettuce, chopped
- 3 ounces grilled chicken or lamb, chopped
- 1/2 cup chopped cucumber
- 1 TBSP diced red onion
- 1 TSP fresh oregano leaves

ARUGULA ASPARAGUS AND CHICKEN SALAD

Ingredients:

- 2 cups arugula
- 3 ounces grilled chicken, chopped
- 5-6 stalks of asparagus, cut into 1" lengths

GINGER AVOCADO POWER DRESSING

- 1/2 cup coconut or olive oil
- 1/3 cup raw apple cider vinegar
- 1/4 cup coconut aminos
- 1/2 cup water
- 2 tablespoon fresh ginger, grated
- 1 avocado

Blend and dress your salad!

SIDE DISHES

FABULOUS KALE CHIPS

Servings: 4

- 1 large bunch of dino kale, stems removed and leaves chopped
- extra virgin olive oil
- sea salt to taste

Massage kale with olive oil, sprinkle with sea salt and bake at 350 for 15 min. Let cool and give thanks for a great snack!

BRAISED GREENS

Servings: 4

- 2 TBSP coconut or olive oil
- 2 heads of greens
- 1/2 yellow onion, chopped
- 3 garlic cloves, chopped
- 1 1/2 cup vegetable, chicken, or beef stock
- Sea salt to taste
- 2 TBSP apple cider vinegar

Sautee onion and garlic until golden brown then add greens, salt, and vinegar. Cover and let the greens cook down for 20 minutes.

SWEET POTATO FRIES

Servings: 4

- 3 medium sweet potatoes, washed and peeled
- 3 TBSP coconut or olive oil
- Sea salt to taste

Coat sweet potatoes with oil and salt. Spread on a baking sheet and bake at 425 degrees for 20 minutes.

CARMELIZED BRUSSELS SPROUTS

Servings: 4

- 1 pound of Brussels sprouts
- 3 TBSP balsamic vinegar
- 3 TBSP olive oil

Sautee sprouts in olive oil on low heat until tender. Increase to high heat and add balsamic vinegar, stirring for 30 seconds. Turn off flame and season with salt to taste.

NORI CHIPS

Servings: 1

- 3 Nori sheets
- Olive oil
- Sea salt to taste

Preheat oven to 350. Cut Nori sheets into four and place on baking sheet. Brush or massage Nori with oil. Add sea salt and whatever spices you choose. Bake for 15 minutes. Let cool.

SAUTEED KALE

Servings: 4

- 2 bunches of kale, leaves pulled off, discard stems
- 2 cloves garlic, finely chopped

- 1 TBSP olive oil

Sautee garlic in olive oil until golden brown, add in kale until tender.

GINGER ROOT TEA

- 4-6 cup filtered water
- 2 TBSP freshly grated ginger root
- 1 TBSP fresh lemon juice

Bring ginger close to boil. Turn off heat and let sit for 5-10 min. Add lemon juice and strain into a cup. You can reuse the ginger more than once by adding more water and heating.

SNACKS

- Cucumber with sea salt
- Herbal tea
- Mixed fruit
- Coconut milk smoothie with plum, nectarine, peach, apple
- Nori Chips
- Kale Chips
- Coconut water kefir
- Coconut yogurt
- Avocado with sauerkraut
- Grated, Carrot, Daikon with Nori
- Bone Broth
- Veggie Broth
- Plaintain chips with avocado
- Jicama sticks with avocado
- Coconut chips

DESSERTS

PALEO BERRY ICE CREAM

Servings: 4

- 1 pint of blueberries or your favorite berries
- 1/2 cup coconut milk
- 1 TSP vanilla extract

Blend everything in food processor and place in freezer.

RASPBERRIES WITH BALSAMIC AND COCONUT MILK

Servings: 2

- 40 raspberries
- 2 TBSP balsamic vinegar
- coconut milk

Cover raspberries in a bowl with 2 TBSP of balsamic and let sit for 15 minutes. Drizzle with coconut milk.

COCONUT YOGURT

1. Heat 1 quart of unsweetened coconut milk to 105F - 110F.
2. Add ¼ teaspoon of yogurt starter and pulse 2x with the blender. You can add more than 1/4 teaspoon per quart if a very firm yogurt is desired.
3. Plug in your yogurt maker and pour the mixture into your yogurt maker container or containers and ferment for 12 hours.
4. Place in refrigerator for 4 hours. Enjoy with blueberries.

SMOOTHIES

GREEN SMOOTHIES

- 1/2 a bunch dino kale or Swiss chard, cut out stalks
- 1/2 inch ginger
- ½ cup blueberries
- 5 cups of water

Blend for 5 minutes.

AIP POWER SHAKE

- 1 Banana
- ½ cup blueberries
- ½ inch ginger
- 1 cup coconut yogurt
- ½ cup coconut milk

Blend for 2 minutes.

ABOUT THE AUTHOR

Anne Angelone, Licensed Acupuncturist

Bachelor of Science, Cornell University

Master of Science, American College of Traditional Chinese Medicine

Member of:

- Primal Docs
- The Paleo Physician's Network
- Dr. Kharrazian's Thyroid Docs

✦ Background ✦

My own experience with Ankylosing Spondylitis (AS) led me to study the underlying mechanisms of disease expression. While learning how to treat AS, which is correlated to the gene type called HLA B-27, I learned how to identify and remove specific triggers and how to heal my leaky gut. Over the course of my exploration, I learned how it's possible to turn off inflammatory gene expression with nutrition, supplements, Qi, acupuncture, exercise, diet, and meditation. I'm grateful to be able to share what I have learned through experience and years of research, training, and investigation.

My path led me to acupuncture school. I also had the opportunity to study the emerging system of Functional Medicine (developed by Dr. Jeffrey Bland), which taught me how to investigate the underlying causes of disease.

Halting AS was a top priority for me, so I have searched high and low for the best, most efficient way to detect the underlying causes of my own autoimmune reactions. I first went gluten-, dairy-, and nightshade-free, and then I went to work on healing my leaky gut, clearing hidden infections, balancing hormones, getting adequate nutrition, and replenishing glutathione.

Over time, and after much additional research, I discovered that a no-starch diet was more appropriate for treating AS, so I was drawn to and inspired by the concepts and science in the field of Paleo Nutrition (with its no-grain, no-legume template). I also learned from the astute teachings about autoimmunity by Dr. Loren Cordain and Robb Wolf, which went further to suggest the elimination of eggs, nuts, seeds, potatoes, eggplants, peppers, and tomatoes. This is a similar template to what Dr. Datis Kharrazian, a leading Functional Medicine practitioner, recommends in his leaky gut repair program. I used this dietary template while following Dr. Kharrazian's Repairvite program and started to improve dramatically.

Soon afterwards, I saw researcher Sarah Ballantyne, Ph.D. report that nightshade- and seed-based spices were also potential leaky gut irritants. When I removed these spices from my diet, I learned how to further control my inflammation. I then collaborated with Dr. Ballantyne to compile an advanced autoimmune protocol list of foods to include/avoid based on evidence in the scientific literature. We indicated whether or not a particular food is immunogenic, allergenic, hard to digest, likely to feed gut bacterial overgrowths, and likely to contribute to leaky gut, dysbiosis, and/or blood sugar imbalances.

This work is important because as of the writing of this book there has been no standardized knowledge base of the herbs, foods, and compounds that are stimulating the imbalanced immune systems of those with autoimmune disease. We also included foods that are potentially problematic (i.e., foods that should be considered as possible triggers if patients are not improving). These foods include FODMAPs and high-histamine, high-salicylate, and high-oxalate foods.

My goal has always been to prevent the decades of suffering that go along with inflammation and untamed autoimmune reactions. I have dedicated my career as an acupuncturist and Functional Medicine practitioner to understanding and teaching about autoimmune triggers and natural medicine solutions for autoimmune disease.

Please help me spread the word about the simple yet profound equation for halting autoimmune reactions—it's all about removing triggers, resolving intestinal permeability (leaky gut), and silencing inflammatory gene expression. By sharing this important information, we can treat the underlying causes of the chronic symptoms experienced by those suffering from autoimmune disease.

Visit my website (www.paleobreakthrough.com) for more information or to find out how to contact me.

Many thanks to the leaders who have inspired me in the fields of Traditional Chinese Medicine, Functional Medicine and Paleo Nutrition: Sarah Ballantyne, Ph.D., Eric Gordon, MD, Kevin Doherty, MS, L.Ac., Dr. Tom O'Bryan, Dr. Terry Wahls, Dr. Deanna Minich, Dr. Jeffrey Bland, Dr. Datis Kharrazian, Dr. Alex Vasquez, Dr. Mark Hyman, Dr. Alison Siebecker, Chris Kresser, MS, L.Ac., Diane Sanfilippo, BS, NC, Robb Wolf, Nora Gegaudas, Dr. Loren Cordain, Mat Lalonde, Ph.D., Dr. Alessio Fasano, Elaine Gottschall, Natasha Campbell McBride, Stephen Wright, and Jordan Reasoner.

Special thanks to Sarah Ballantyne, Ph.D. aka The Paleo Mom for support, guidance and inspiration in writing The Autoimmune Paleo Breakthrough.

I am proud to say that this book has been officially approved by Dr. Ballantyne and The Paleo Approach.

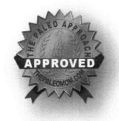

ADDITIONAL RESOURCES

OTHER BOOKS ABOUT AUTOIMMUNE DISEASE
BY ANNE ANGELONE

- The FODMAP Free Paleo Breakthrough
- The Paleo Autoimmune Protocol

AUTOIMMUNE RESOURCES

- The Paleo Approach &
- The Paleo Approach Cookbook
  by Sarah Ballantyne, Ph.D.
- Dr. Ballantyne's website: ThePaleoMom.com
- Autoimmune, Clean Eating and You
- Autoimmune-Paleo.com
- The Autommune Paleo Cookbook
  by Mickie Trescott
- Practical Paleo by Diane Sanfilippo
- Chris Kresser's: Personal Paleo Code
- The Paleo Parents Pinterest page
- Dr. Datis Kharrazian's Brain and Thyroid Books
- Thepaleoplan.com
- CyrexLabs.com

The Paleo Approach: Reverse Autoimmune Disease and Heal Your Body by Sarah Ballantyne, PhD.

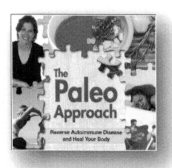

29834136R00069

Made in the USA
Lexington, KY
13 February 2014